Living Healthy at 50

and Beyond

Robert Howe

Living Healthy at 50 and Beyond
Robert Howe

Table of Contents

For My Father, Ralph D. Howe, MD

Ralph Howe came to the peninsula from Iowa with a family of nine plus his parents. His dad was a contractor who helped build Stanford University. His dad's dream was to send his children to Stanford University.

Ralph Howe went to Palo Alto High School and then attended Stanford University. Upon graduation he was accepted to Stanford University Medical School. One of his brothers went to Law School at Stanford University. Three others went to Dental School. So his father's dream was partially realized. One of Ralph Howe's sisters married a mining engineer who graduated from Stanford University.

Ralph Howe married his high school sweetheart who became a teacher and school principal. She helped him through medical school. No scholarships for medical school were available at the time. Dr. Howe came to Redwood City and opened an office for a General Medical Practice.

He continued to take advanced medical classes well into his fifties. In one of our discussions he told me a medical doctor could never know enough about the human anatomy and how it functions. This book is dedicated to him and is partially built upon a large sampling of his

4

medical cases. We spent many enjoyable times discussing both physical

and psychological aspects of medicine. This book will present this

man's practical health realities to you the reader.

Chapter 1: Introduction

Most medical equations deal with illness and its resolution. Too often wellness is often a neglected issue. Yet this is where medical providers should be putting in their best efforts. Too often when illness is first observed its treatment is normally complicated. Had the focus been on wellness in the first place there might not have arisen any illness issues at all. Such common concerns as high blood pressure, overweight, Type II Diabetes and other normally occurring health issues might easily have been avoided.

My father who was a physician for over 50 years would certainly have agreed with the above proposition that wellness should be the major focus for both the physician and the patient. In going over some 10,000 of his patient's medical records it was apparent that despite Dr. Howe's expertise as a medical diagnostician, illness issues over time became apparent in his long-term patients. The question always arose, "Why was this happening?" I am sure it was an issue that involved both the patient and the physician. For the most part Dr. Howe could see illness over-coming his patients as they went through the gradual aging process. Most of his patients were with him for a considerable period of time and this gave him a great advantage in viewing the aging and illness process as it developed over this lengthy time span. He became most familiar with the habits and characteristics of his long-term patients.

Too often as a skilled physician he could easily see various illnesses looming over the horizon for many of his patients. Often he would make suggestions to them that would require them to change some of their ingrained habit patterns. Some illnesses can be a long-term process that does not become a full bloom reality for some time.

Such procedures can often be halted by making changes in certain ingrained personal habits. We can see many examples of this quite easily. Many of them come to mind such as smoking, drinking of alcoholic beverages in excess, weight gain over time, a lack of proper nutrition and far too little exercise. This list can be quite exhaustive yet all of such habits can easily be monitored and detected by any competent physician or by a specialist. Properly handled these above issues need not be an occasion for any alarm or concern over the possibility of serious health issues arising.

Too often major problems may arise simply because the patient or even the doctor might ignore such recurring issues in the here and now that could reasonably be taken care of quite easily over time.

As my dad said so often to me in our discussions on health and wellness issues that he could easily put "10 to 20" years on the life expectancies of his patients if he could only convince them to undertake certain practical health practices. Perhaps this book will help obtain these extra 10 or 20 years for you!

Too often Dr. Howe would become frustrated that his patients would either ignore certain obvious health practices or very much like new years resolutions they would simply begin to fail to adopt the proper health suggestions made by him and revert back to some of their old destructive ways.

He would become quite frustrated that patients would often have all sorts of excuses for failing to follow 'doctor's orders.' Just a few examples are illustrative of these problems. For example failing to stay on a proper medical diet, not taking blood pressure readings on a regular basis or a failure to start and continue a regular exercise program or not observing a proper diet in a systematic fashion. These and many other failures to observe basic health practices over time often led to illnesses of various types that could have been easily avoided.

An issue that is particularly ugly yet often ignored or neglected is that of high blood pressure. It is a most common ailment and yet one that can be particularly dangerous. Many millions of Americans presently suffer <u>unknowingly</u> from this disorder. This is particularly so since in its beginning high blood pressure demonstrates few if any medical symptoms. Some may think it will simply go away or others may simply be unaware that they have the disorder or that they feel it is harmless.

This very "silent killer" can unfortunately produce over some time very ugly disorders. These may include heart disease, kidney failure and even very debilitating strokes. This latter disorder may easily disable people or it may cause premature death in the prime of their life. While the condition of high blood pressure is often hazardous to your health it can ironically be easily treated. High blood pressure is or has both organic and external origins. Even though you may have a genetic issue affecting your blood pressure often other factors may be influential ones that can be controlled. These include such issues as undo stress, improper diet, and lack of exercise and overuse of alcohol and or tobacco. However people who suffer from chronic high blood pressure issues can with minor life style changes keep destructive health issues associated with this condition under control. For example members of my own family had concerns regarding the occurrence of high blood pressure. Among our family salt sodium sensitivity was an issue. Living on a low sodium diet for a lifetime could do much to resolve this potential problem. Unfortunately, unresolved issues such as this condition can lead to serious health consequences. By way of example two of my relatives died prematurely by neglecting their blood pressure or similarly related issues.

It is vitally important that the patient should take on an active role in dealing with health issues that the physician detects in his diagnosis. Here in lies the rub of the medical dilemma. The physician may not be trained in presenting his findings <u>correctly</u> to the patient or the individual may see his problems as a death sentence that they can do nothing about. The patient may think, "My father died of that or my brother had a similar particular disorder and could do nothing about it." Perhaps the physician after failed attempts to convince the patient may simply choose to quit trying to evoke the desired changes from the patient. A most notably unresolved medical issue is dieting. Time and again the patient may attempt dieting but the result often ends in failure.

Presently there are healthy life style programs like weight management and eat healthy programs that physicians and patients can utilize to help reach their more desired health goals. Physicians should continue to encourage patients to lose weight and help maintain a healthy weight. You may want to check with your own private physician to see what programs are available to you. The success of weight loss, to a great extent, is patient driven, and should have a high level of motivation from the individual patient. Unfortunately there is only so much a doctor can do if the patient is not motivated or willing to change their lifestyle. Even prescription weight loss drugs have limitations.

For the physician the most difficult thing to overcome is the individual patient's long ingrained habit patterns. For example some physicians have claimed that the cessation of smoking is often more difficult to give up than the issues of alcohol abuse or narcotics addition.

So how can this dilemma of communication blockage in medical information and patient behavior be resolved? There are a number of things that can or should be done! First there needs to be more effective communication between the doctor and the patient. A book of this nature should be of some help! The more knowledge the patient has about health issues the more likely he or she will ask their doctor better informed questions. Then the doctor can provide specific information to their patients.

As previously stated many HMOs provide classes that help inform their members about issues of proper health practices. Classes are often offered on such subjects as diabetes, stress reduction, weight loss and diet, proper exercise approaches and many other important health related issues. The HMOs are indeed finding that more informed patients make for much healthier and happier individuals. Nevertheless both patients and physicians must learn how to communicate effectively with each other.

The information they hold between them must be shared and utilized for the benefit of both parties plus the families that may be involved. The ultimate goal then is for an effective shared communication system that will bring about long and lasting health for all concerned. Finally such a medical information delivery program second to none can be achieved over time. Hopefully this small book may well add to the knowledge of all concerned: doctors, patient's family members and the total medical establishment. So may your further reading of this work add to your good future health outlook.

Chapter 2: Your Weight and its Effective Control

More than 72 million US adults now face the situation of being obese. The medical care cost due to obesity is about 14 billion in total a year. Being overweight in America is indeed a major public health issue. Being in this condition will often lead to serious medical problems. Recent research findings reported by the Wall Street Journal (May 3, 2011) underscores the importance of proper diet and especially physical exercise in combating overweight conditions particularly those concerning belly fat.

The WSJ article goes on to suggest that people with enlarged waistlines carry a much greater risk of having a heart attack than people with normal waistlines. The reported study indicates that belly fat in particular is a major factor involved in obesity and the developing of cardiovascular disease. Researchers reveal that belly fat releases toxins that can adversely effect your blood vessels and then finally your heart.

While being overweight must be controlled it is patients with bulging waistlines as measured by their waist circumference or waist to hip ratios who have a much higher risk of death. These groups were 1.7 times more likely to die during a follow up than those with normal waistline measurements. A waistline measurement for men more than 40 inches and women more than 35 inches are considered to be in the danger zone. This WSJ article looked at patients who had suffered a heart attack or had a major heart procedure. Other large studies also have suggested that belly fat is related to a higher risk of heart attacks and other heart and blood vessel issues.

Every year in the United States alone some 300,000 or more adults die from causes partly related to excessive body weight. Being in this condition normally is often the result of taking in more food or calories than we use up in the course of a day. The headline on the above cited WSJ article shouted, "The Bigger the Belly the Bigger the Risk."

A person is considered overweight or obese when their weight is greater than what is considered healthy for a given height. A person is obese when their weight is 20% above what is considered normal weight. Body mass index (BMI) is a marker that is used to calculate overweight and obesity. A BMI of 25 to 29.9 is considered overweight and 30 or higher is considered obese. This measurement is calculated by dividing your weight in kilograms by your height in meters squared. Although there are genetic and hormonal influences on body weight normally weight gain occurs when you take in more calories than you burn. The true key to weight loss is healthy eating, portion control and calorie reduction. In the beginning of a diet, it may be helpful to keep a food and activity journal. This will allow you to see your food consumption

14

and activities level. The American College of Sports Medicine recommends for individuals to lose weight you should get at least 150 minutes a week of moderate exercise.

Remember if you're not very active you don't burn as many calories. Remember also that obesity based on eating habits tends to run in families. Questions when checking body weight with a physician are the following, "Why can't I overcome obesity on my own? What treatment options should I consider?" The physician can and will point you in the right direction to weight loss.

Being overweight particularly over time increases the risk of developing a significant number of serious medical conditions such as coronary heart disease, Type II Diabetes, high cholesterol, abnormal blood pressure, breathing disorders during sleep, some types of cancer, osteoarthritis, urinary problems and many other disturbing health conditions. This list can be seen as quite exhaustive.

It is too simplistic to say that overweight conditions are caused by overeating. Unfortunately in one sense this is a brutal truism. So what can be done about this apparent simplistic issue? Just like smoking, should we say, "Stop smoking!" And for over eating, should we just say, "Stop eating so much!" Unfortunately both of these apparently simple conditions are not so easily resolved by the individual without a considerable amount of personal will power and expert help!

The average American may often put on as much as 40 pounds between the ages of 20 and 40 years of age. This seems to be a horrendous amount of weight to put on overtime and it is indeed the case!

As a result of this possibility we must have a keen awareness of healthy eating habits and proper physical activities early on. All the better that we might curb or prevent such weight gain which is so often difficult to eliminate once it is put on our bodies. This is certainly important for all adults and not just for those who are already overweight or obese. That is why it is vitally important to have sufficient knowledge to make wise food choices and to learn to stay active in a way that will contribute to our overall health. Your good health should always be a lifetime concern of yours. You normally will properly maintain a car and it will respond by performing better over an extended lifetime. The same is true of your body; keep the body well tuned for a lifetime and it will serve the owner well. Long life expectancy is not an accident.

There are a variety of reasons weight-loss diets normally do not work well. The doctor may not present weight loss and dieting in an effective and appealing manner. Patients may have experienced failure many times in this area and they simply are not willing to try again. Further, it is important to remember that food generally may be a strong reinforcer to a person for many reasons. Food is often seen as a positive

16

form of a reward system. Food is also a strong part of our social interactions as well. Our lives have become so hectic that it is difficult to cook everyday. As an alternative to this we eat out and often the food is high in fat and salt products.

As we get older and become less active it is important to consider decreasing our food consumption. Furthermore it is equally important to incorporate healthy food choices into our meals. Healthy eating can give you more energy, help you lose weight and live a longer and healthier life.

Culturally as a nation we have become less labor intensive, fewer people are working hard on the farms and ranches. Though our work may be less physically active our eating habits may not have changed. For example my grandfather was a carpenter contractor who worked 10 to 14 hours a day, six days a week and he lived to be 89 years old. This is despite the fact that his diet consisted primarily of meat, potatoes and gravy. Yet he never experienced any weight problems or major health issues.

Habits of over-eating or incorrect eating are often very hard to change. Diets may often make us feel somewhat deprived. Food as suggested can be powerful reinforces. For example, in animal training, trainers use food as a reward. The overweight issue can sting anyone, anywhere. I am a perfect example of just such a condition. Even the so-called experts fall prey to weight issues in their life.

For example when playing college football I was in excellent condition. At 6'3" I weighed 214 lbs and was all muscle. The work schedule was hard. Conditioning programs were twice a day! With this much exercise I was eating three large meals a day and not gaining an ounce of weight. After football season I did gain some weight but dropped down once training started again.

Upon graduating I worked as a teacher and coached and continued to exercise regularly. Unfortunately I kept eating those big meals of the past when playing football and thus my weight slowly crept up. Then I became an administrator and my physical activity level went down and my weight continued to escalate. Before I knew it my once athletic body didn't look that way anymore. I surprised myself by getting on the scale one day and saw the number 255 appear. I was totally shocked! But not enough to stop eating those large football induced meals. I thought to myself, "This is easy I'll just exercise more." Unfortunately this was not much help. I was ignorant of calorie counting and proper nutrition issues. As with so many other people my weight over time unfortunately kept going up and down. This of course is not healthy for your body.

This is something that happens to all of us unfortunately we gain weight unknowingly and often times out of a state of ignorance. Once weight goes on your body it is extremely difficult to take off, permanently. Bad habits are difficult to change. Often the weight simply returns after you have lost some surplus flesh.

I am an example of the old truism that fad diets just don't work. Unfortunately it was true in my case, as it is the case for so many others. It is easy to simply throw the towel in and just simply give up. Most of us have made some of these comments, "Well I am a big person. I eat very little but I seem to gain weight. Why should I deprive myself? I just don't have the will power. Almost everyone around me is over weight. My doctor looks pretty out of shape and that doesn't seem to bother him." The human mind is often very inventive, particularly as we get older and the need to have a fit body becomes perhaps less paramount in our personal lives. Eventually unhealthy eating and bad habits will catch up with you. Certain irritating and unpleasant health issues begin to arise, for example high blood pressure, heart disease, or pre-diabetes.

In my case I was very fortunate to get off the weight rollercoaster. My very smart and loving wife, a fine medical doctor, a couple of good health books and an expert nutritionist contributed to the solution for me. I found the right information and my approach was to apply it over my lifetime. It was not easy but well worth the effort. I am now 214 lbs (my old football weight in college) and have been that way for years. The equation was simple, eat healthy and exercise regularly. The execution was more difficult, but with time and a lot of self-discipline I started to shed the extra pounds. With continual effort I have been able to keep my current weight.

The important thing as it is in so many vital issues you must not give up until success has been achieved. Failure is not an option. It is important to remember that in most worthwhile projects you may have to go through any number of failure modes. Whether that's being a good student, a strong athlete or a good cook you will always experience some setbacks. But please don't let failure curb your normal resolve; rather persevere. The key is to get expert help and keep at it. Without this mind set it will be a very difficult road to a proper weight goal. It is one of those things that are unfortunately both easily worthwhile and yet hard or elusive to achieve.

Often there are so many programs dealing with weight loss that it can be daunting. So we arbitrary pick one or we may stay away from any expert help completely. The important thing to remember is that something must be done sooner or later. Otherwise the consequences can be devastating to your health.

One consequence is heart surgery. Heart surgery is not a cure all. It is important for patients to incorporate a healthy life style after surgery. Yet unfortunately medical studies have shown that 2 years after surgery 90% of the patients have not alter their life styles. On the surface it seems that most would rather die than change! How stupid can a person be? Weight loss will naturally come when the right food choices are made. Remember with reasonable discipline and some information you may be able to save your own life. It is after all up to you and you alone!

One caveat should be remembered; crash diets will normally not work. So avoid them if at all possible. A slow steady change to a new and long-term life style is the best way to go. As you progress one should use both short-term and long-term goal setting, often using support groups along the way! Join a gym, try the buddy system, and join a well-recognized weight loss program. There are indeed many varied ways to get this important job done. Just remember it is hard to do it all by yourself. Just will power doesn't always work that well.

One problem often impeding success is the failure to use a scale on a regular basis. Ignorance is not bliss, you need to discipline yourself on a daily, weekly, monthly, life time basis or most of your best efforts will turn out to be fruitless. Just look at all the overweight populations here and abroad. Believe me most of them despite rationalizations to the contrary do not like carrying all the extra weight they now own.

To be sure about your final fitness level all one needs to do is consult one or more of the insurance companies statistical charts. After all they are experts on weight control. They have all sorts of statisticians that know exactly what you should weigh. They are paid big money to be right about your correct weight. Their company's profits depend upon accuracy in this statistical arena!

One last comment about your weight issue, you don't have to be paranoid about it. A few pounds one way or the other will not cause a major health issue. Just get it done regularly for a lifetime! You should then be a happy camper. If you are overly obsessed about weight control this can turn into a difficult and unnecessary issue in your life. Please do remember that your medical doctor should be a key individual for you in this battle of the bulge!

Here are some issues you should follow up on. Ask your doctor for any diet plans he/she recommends. Also ask for educational brochures on eating correctly, calorie counting, and physical activity programs that may be available to you. In addition request to have your BMI calculated and ask your doctor what it means in regards to your health status. Have your waist circumference measured and discuss its health significance with your doctor. Be prepared to discuss in detail your current diet and activity levels and what changes need to be made for health reasons. Do think about how much change you are willing to make. Ask about access to health specialists available to you in your medical plan, people such as dieticians, nutritionist, physical trainers, etc. Once again remember that like anything else in life, "That by the inch change is a cinch but by the yard things are indeed most difficult!"

While failure rates among diets are quite high many popular ones do seem to work. However if you lose weight drastically it will be difficult to keep it off. For this reason it is so important for you to find healthy food choices that you actually like and physical activities that you may genuinely enjoy for a life time. In my own life I have experienced my ups and downs in dieting. Without solid and genuine caring help you too will be on the yo-yo weight trip! Too often after a while many people simply give up! This is something you must not be trapped into for the rest of your life! Unfortunately, I fell into this trap three times. Finally I hit the right combinations. Often to get it right requires serious warnings from your doctor. Or perhaps a loved one can pressure you in the right way. Or you may hit on a procedure that fits your own particular needs. The most important thing is not to quit or give up. Particularly do not quit because of some stupid personal rationalizations. I just have big bones. It is my genetic inheritance, my mother was that way and she lived to be 80 years old. Do not fall into these death traps or others. You must keep at it until you truly overcome. Remember it is your good health and that alone should be worth enough as a major motivator. Remember with excess weight comes unwanted heart attacks, strokes, bad knees and any number of other unwanted events that can cause physical debilitation or cut short your life unnecessarily.

The joy of family and friends can often disappear under the onslaught of undesirable health consequences from being permanently overweight. Do remember that going through heart surgery is not a fun option to undergo.

You are not alone in the overweight condition. The Center of Disease Control and Prevention in the United States reports overweight is the number one health concern in America. In other words it is vitally important to you and many others that we deal with this disorder in some detail! Not only for your sake but for all the millions of other Americas also suffering from overweight issues.

When my dad was older and in his reflective state he told me something most important. He stated, "Many people see me as very smart." I certainly did! "But Bob I found that whatever I set my mind to do, I could accomplished it." In essence he was saying that a little will power can and will go a long way! Perhaps we pooh-poohed the natural instincts of man. Will power is indeed a natural instinct and we should not ignore it. Particularly when we can team this with great medical services, work out facilities and expert nutritional resources presently available to us.

What for the most part has caused this nation wide explosion in overweight conditions in America? I believe a simple example from my family may illustrate the growth of the problem. As mentioned before my paternal grandfather was a hardworking carpenter contractor. He worked at hard physical labor some 10 to 14 hours a day, six days a week. In addition he built his own family house and also three rental units. He fell off a roof at 70 something while he was repairing it and yet lived to be 89 years old. This is despite the fact that his diet often consisted of meat and potatoes. For obvious reasons he was never overweight. His wife had nine children and she did her own housework. Indeed a hardworking family. All nine of their children went to college and were soon doing white collar and professional work.

This next generation was involved primarily in mental work and thus did little physical labor. So this group was somewhat overweight and their progeny did the same line of work as their parents and ate out quite frequently. Thus less pure physical labor brings on weight gain over time.

Yet another sedentary activity adding to the weight gain issue is the addition of more and better cars. We drive our cars for most if not all errands even if we could and would have the time to walk instead we choose to drive. Then topping this off is the sudden advent of television. Both children and adults presently are literally watching too many hours of television. We also have added sedentary activities such as, video games, computers, internet, and reading instead of outdoor activities, such as, golfing, tennis, hiking, biking, running, jogging, walking, gardening etc. All these issues have brought on us the "couch potato syndrome" and a true weight gain explosion. The rise of weight gain has become the harsh reality of modern day America! Add to this is the reality that hard work on the farms and ranches have disappeared. For these reasons we must incorporate physical activity into our daily lives.

Populations were rushing to the cities for less labor-intensive jobs. White collar was now the way to go, both for status and the money it provided. Rather than labor intensive work the reality became desk jobs and computer terminals. So here we are now in a new reality. Work is presently no longer physical labor and demanding for most of us. My grandfather never had to worry about his weight, my father as a doctor did and I as a psychologist definitely had much more severe weight problems. Discussing mental health issues with patients is definitely mental not physical activity based work.

So in a generation or two we have created our own major health problems – overweight conditions and their related serious health issues.

26

So now it is up to us in this generation to solve this high level problem or it will become a health problem or rather a disaster to this generation and this country and to you and your immediate family. This is so important that individually and collectively we must solve this calamity that has been brought on by a dynamic and yet problematic society. The doctors can't solve it alone it must be an individual and collective effort to solve this most serious and epidemic problem. So let's work together to resolve yet another problem that has hit our shore like some giant tidal wave that hopefully will not sweep us into a national disaster.

One last comment should be made relative to our weight issues. We all have a hard time viewing harsh truths on a daily or weekly basis yet facts are facts and we need to use them effectively in controlling our own weight issues.

My wife illustrates proper weight control by watching her weight. First she has an approximate number of pounds she wishes to weigh. On a daily basis she trudges to the bathroom and jumps on the scale to read her weight. If it is off a bit she adjusts her eating habits and physical activity accordingly and the scale returns to an established and positive norm. She is not obsessed about weight control and she does enjoy good food. But this little habit has kept her fit and her blood pressure well controlled. I, on the other hand, was not so well disciplined and as a result my weight would get out of bounds along with my blood pressure. Luckily I have learned this little habit of discipline from her and am now a happy camper! So follow this little trick and you will also be a happy health addict!

Chapter 3: Your Blood Pressure

Blood pressure improperly supervised can be a strong and yet silent killer, just like an overweight condition. Both fortunately can be easily controlled. For example, you should have a simple blood pressure machine available so that you can keep track of your blood pressure either on a daily or weekly basis.

If your blood pressure is a little high seek counsel from your doctor and more than likely it can be controlled without drugs, particularly if caught early. High blood pressure often produces no obvious conspicuous symptoms. Unfortunately if left undiagnosed your condition can easily slip into a state of hypertension that may have to be controlled by drug therapy. So here we have two simple medical devices (scales and blood pressure device), properly used they can really help give you a healthy body with only minimum effort on your part.

For example my life was saved by mere happenstance. I made a visit to the dentist's office and luckily for me she monitored all her patients on blood pressure issues! My blood pressure was high so she suggested I have it retaken by my primary care physician. When my blood pressure was taken at the doctor's office again it registered high and I was placed on medication, which luckily for me controlled the condition. Later with hard work by eating a low sodium and low fat diet and increasing my physical activity I no longer need the medication.

As you can see a high blood pressure condition can literally sneak up on you. You certainly don't want to depend on luck for your health. Weight control and proper blood pressure treatment are closely related and so important for your health. Both are somewhat easily controlled with basic discipline on your part. Between weight and blood pressure issues you are probably dealing with at least 50% of your potential health issues. Please take these three chapters seriously. They will do so much for your long-term health and longevity.

Many experts label high blood pressure as the number one cause of death in the United States. In the US alone approximately 45 to 50 million men and women suffer from this silent killer. That is approximately 20% of the adult population in the US.

As we age older individuals are more likely to experience hypertension than are younger individuals. For example it is reported more than 60% of people in there 60's have blood pressure above the normal range. So with aging often comes some elevation in blood pressure.

Blood pressure related to heredity is a most interesting issue. If one of your parents has hypertension your chances of getting this disorder is about 50/50. If both parents have it this increases your chances even more so. For example my father was hypertensive but not my mother. My father passed on this genetic information of sodium sensitivity to me. However my father passed on invaluable medical information that helped me immeasurable. He told me I must control my salt intake and exercise regularly. It turned out to be the truth. As a result of watching my sodium intake and proper exercise my blood pressure is now relatively low.

So we do know that blood pressure is often affected by our life styles. So certain life style factors are often determinants in high blood pressure issues. It must, however be remembered that your blood pressure rises and falls during the day depending on what you are doing. A constant heighten blood pressure however can affect the hardening of the arteries and is thus dangerous and may start the road towards a possible stroke.

Please do remember that according to many medical authorities one in three strokes can be fatal! So our blood pressure is an important issue to take care of immediately and in the long term. Fortunately if caught in time hardening of the arteries is to some degree reversible. This can be accomplished through the use of medication, proper diet, exercise and lifestyle changes.

A very famous study should be mentioned here to show that there is a strong relationship between high blood pressure and weight;

two key elements in a strong health progression for you. This study is the Framingham Heart Research program which demonstrated that men and women who are 20% above their ideal body weight have eight times greater chance of suffering heightened blood pressure than those who are at their true normal body weight. Those people suffering borderline or mild hypertension often discover they can with weight loss easily reduce their blood pressure to a level of normalcy.

Stroke occurs when an artery in the brain bursts or becomes clogged by a blood clot thus cutting off the supply of oxygen to some part of the brain. Deprived of oxygen the brain tissue often dies within minutes. The body controlled by these damaged brain cells cannot function properly.

Neurological exams can usually confirm a diagnosis for strokes. Drugs can often help prevent new clots from forming or prevent existing clots from getting bigger.

Symptoms of a stroke may include sudden weakness in body parts, a loss of speech, loss of vision, sudden and severe headaches, unexplained dizziness and unsteadiness causing the individual to fall suddenly. Such falls, particularly with the elderly can be harmful. A baby aspirin taken daily can be a positive preventive measure.

How does one normally avoid a stroke? Again a major risk factor is often high blood pressure. You should eat a well balance diet low in cholesterol and saturated fats. If you have diabetes, keep it well controlled, because it is linked to increase risks for strokes. If you smoke, you must quit and use alcohol only in moderation. Any sign of a stroke should be quickly treated since damage can be limited by proper and quick medical intervention.

Another issue effecting blood pressure besides weight gain is stress. Stress is quite common in our hardworking and pressure related society. You and I have often heard of type A and B personalities. The first are primarily people who are aggressive, impatient, often quickly frustrated, easily angered and are according to some authorities perhaps twice as likely to suffer from various heart problems.

Circulatory problems are normally related to type A personalities. Those in the type B category do not have such tendencies at such high levels. For many people then stress at the higher levels can also be a key factor in cardiovascular health. By applying relaxation techniques and medication you can bring high blood pressure levels down to more manageable or normal levels.

Often people with high blood pressure levels have a combination of factors such as over-weight; moderate to high chronic alcohol consumption, and significant stress levels. Fortunately several of these conditions can be diagnosed by a good physician and then treated as a group of issues most successfully!

Many Americans due to their socially imposed life styles often do not get adequate amounts of exercise. In earlier days exercise came right along with your work. Not so in this high tech society in which we live in today.

As far as our own bodies are concerned disuse is a form of health abuse. Unfortunately too many of us in this society are not conditioned to exercise regimes. At some point in time a lack of exercise will normally show up as high blood pressure readings and weight gains particularly as we get older. Unfortunately too often people start regular workout routines and then often abandon them.

Fortunately our present open society does provide a wide assortment of exercise opportunities. These include walking, jogging, running, biking, hiking, golfing and swimming, etc. If at all possible join a workout facility. They offer many classes for cardio exercise, muscle strengthening and training, stretching, and relaxation classes, and more. The facility usually has trainers to help you get started correctly.

The important thing is we must not continue living a couch potato existence. Too many of us permanently occupy this status already. The key however is not just exercise, but regularly done workouts and with some degree of reasonable vigor. Our body over many generations has evolved into a machine. It must be properly maintained.

Fortunately a proper diet may also be one of your greatest assets in the battle against hypertension and weight control. Part of our dietary concerns deal with how much to eat, when and of what quality. Breakfast is the most important meal of the day. According to the Mayo Clinic, when you skip breakfast you prolong the fasting (during your sleep time) and this can increase your insulin response which increases fat storage and leads to weight gain. When you eat breakfast you are on track to make healthy food choices the rest of the day. Eating breakfast refuels your body and replenishes the glycogen stores that supply your muscles. Then you feel more energized and are more physically active during the day.

It is important not to skip meals because that leads to increase insulin response then increase fat storage then weight gain. Healthy food choices, portion control and exercise are key to weight loss and weight management.

One part of our diet that we should monitor to a great extent is our salt intake. Most of the salt we eat comes from packaged store-bought and restaurant food. It is the sodium in the salt compound that induces factors leading to high blood pressure. The dietary guidelines recommend eating 2300mg/day. If you have high blood pressure or chronic kidney disease you should reduce the intake to 1500mg/day. The average American ages 2 and up consume 3,400mg/day. Our bodies only need 180-500mg of sodium per day (CDC). What effect does all this extra sodium have on our bodies?

Extra salt in the body usually causes an increase in water build up in our systems. The volume of blood in our body then increases and causes a rise in our blood pressure. For example in New Foundland a diet of salty fish produces a general population with a high mean average in their blood pressure. A portion of the world's population is definitely more salt sensitive and Americans in particular do fall into this salt sensitive category. It has been found that in some salt sensitive hypertensive people sodium reduction alone can help normalize their blood pressure. Do remember that salt is used in products for taste and preservation so read labels when shopping for food. Additionally, as we grow older our kidneys normally became much less efficient in filtering salt. This gives us another good reason why people over 50 should watch their daily intake of salt.

A major truth in maintaining a restricted salt diet is learning the salt contents of our everyday foods. For example your favorite cakes and pies are loaded with salt laden chemicals most often used for preservation of food products. Frozen dinners are loaded with salt and salt derived chemicals. Here are some other common salt loaded foods bread and rolls, cold cuts and cured meats, pizza, cheese snacks, potato chips, canned soup, tomato juice, commercial macaroni cheese, spaghetti with meat sauce, soy sauce, cucumber pickles, potato salad and sauerkraut.

Always assume when shopping that canned and processed foods do contain many salt bearing additives. Also read all types of medicines, many items such as laxatives, aspirin, antacids, cough medicines and sedatives, may often contain large amounts of salt.

What things should we avoid for better blood pressure readings? We often drink too much alcohol and often eat food high in salt, sugars and fats. As a result of poor nutritional habits all these violations do add up.

A common truism is that health begins and ends in the stomach. While not a food it is apparent that smoking also contributes to a variety of fatal cardiovascular disorders. This would of course include heightened blood pressure. According to the American Heart Association the single most important step you can take to keep your heart sound is not to smoke.

Alcohol is another example of improper eating. We know for certain that <u>alcohol stimulates the hormone cortisol</u>. Increased amounts of this chemical often triggers salt retention and potassium loss in the body. These create reactions for someone suffering from hypertension.

Cholesterol loaded foods can also do negative things to our blood pressure by creating plaque build up in blood vessels thus robbing them of their basic flexibility. These deposits in our vessels can become so large they may slow blood flow, thus elevating the blood pressure in your system. There are two types of cholesterol, HDL (High Density Lipoproteins) and LDL (Low Density Lipoproteins). HDL cholesterol takes the bad cholesterol out of your blood and keeps it from building up in your arteries. This is the reason this cholesterol is considered the "good" cholesterol and the higher the number the lower your risk. The LDL cholesterol can build up on the walls of your arteries and increase your chance of getting heart disease. This is the reason why LDL cholesterol is considered the "bad" cholesterol and the lower the number the lower your risk. The optimal numbers for total cholesterol is less than 200, HDL is 60 and above, LDL less than 100.

It is important to remember that there is no cholesterol in plant foods, such as fruits, vegetables, or grains. It is also to be remembered that our body alone produces some 60 – 70% of our cholesterol, hopefully primarily the good kinds.

Some of the following foods are considered to be heavy in cholesterol: eggs, butter, pound cake, ice cream, cheese, lamb, beef, chicken, whole milk, crab, organ meats, oysters, pork, shrimp, and squid. Generally speaking it is animal fat that people with hypertension are well advised to monitor, control and stay away from large amounts.

Beans for example, are particularly good substitutes for meat. Also include fish once or twice a week. Also bean curd (tofu) makes an excellent meat stand-in. When possible avoid fried foods, particularly deep-fried foods. Also use unsaturated vegetable oils such as canola, olive safflower, corn and soybean oil. Stick to low-fat desserts such as fruits. Also limit your egg count. Generally include no more than 20% fats in your diet. The other 80% should come from protein, fruits, vegetables and carbohydrates.

The intake of potassium has a positive diuretic effect on your body's fluid levels. Too little potassium promotes excess water retention and thus increased levels in your blood pressure. A fairly high level of potassium in your systems tends to keep your blood pressure down. Potassium is especially present in fruits, beans, fish, meat, seeds and whole grains. Examples of high potassium foods are apricots, bananas, avocados, wheat bran, flounder, salmon, chicken, peanuts and sunflower seeds.

Two other elements may help our blood pressure. Magnesium works in direct partnership with calcium by relaxing the body's long strands of muscles while calcium stimulates them and thus help in constricting and relaxing the blood vessels. Foods, especially rich in magnesium are: almonds, bananas, milk and peas.

It should be indicated that some hypertensive drugs especially those in the diuretic class depletes the body of minerals such as potassium, magnesium and calcium. This depletion can exert harmful effects on blood pressure. A high dietary fiber diet might also be helpful and produce a positive effect on your blood pressure.

Countries which diets are rich in fiber almost invariably have low rates of hypertension and atherosclerosis than is found in the industrialized economies. The benefit of fiber is that it encourages weight loss and proper bowel movements, lowers cholesterol levels and helps control blood sugar level. High fiber foods include apples, avocados, wheat bran, broccoli, lentil soup parsnip, pineapple, prunes and spinach.

A number of studies indicate that eating fish just twice a week has been found to reduce the risk of heart attacks by as much as 25 to 50%. Fish which are rich in omega -3-fatty acids appear to be the ones effective in lowering blood pressure for people with mild hypertension. More than 60 double blind studies have indicated lower blood pressure and lower cholesterol levels for people using fish oil on a consistent basis. Just don't overdo it. Daily doses of niacin also lower blood cholesterol and raises the "good"HDL. One should eat a nutrient rich diet and avoid vitamin-depleting habits such as smoking, drinking, and drug taking and that one should also take a good vitamin supplement once a day.

The best or a reasonable diet for hypertension is summed up by a study done in 1994 research labeled DASH or Dietary Approaches to Stop Hypertension. The study was carried out on 459 adult men and women by the National Heart Lung and Blood Institute. Its purpose was to determine whether blood pressure could be reduced by a diet based on whole foods rather than individual nutrients. The study subjects were based on high, normal and mild high blood pressure individuals. These were people with systolic readings below 160mmhg and diastolic readings between 80 and 95mmHg. They were assigned one of three diets to take during an eight-week period. The third diet produced the best results. It contained meals rich in vegetables, fruits, and one low in saturated fat and total fat adding up to 27% of total calorie consumption. Subjects on this regime experience an average blood pressure drop of 5.5 points systolic and 3 points diastolic. Subjects with mild hypertension on the above diet showed blood pressure drops of an average 11 points, systolic and 5.5 diastolic.

The DASH dieters were advised to lower fat intake and plan meals around rice, beans, pasta and vegetables rather than meat protein. A Harvard researcher indicated that the potassium content of the diet pretty much explains why it lowered blood pressure. Potassium might foster sodium excretion from the body! The researcher further contends that calcium and magnesium, which are also heavy in this diet, are effective in lowering blood pressure. There are many other combinations of diets that can be effective and are readily available in the literature.

Along with this news is the good news that high blood pressure is eminently treatable. Many factors influence your blood pressure. These can include undue stress, improper diet, and lack of exercise; over use of alcohol, poor weight control and tobacco usage will all take their toll. So people who suffer blood pressure problems perhaps all that is needed for you is a reasonable lifestyle change.

All we need to do is to take and seriously consider lifestyle tools that are already available to us in the commonly read literature. Fundamentally then the choice is yours. It is a simple one! Read the literature, inform yourself, find a quality physician who cares about your health and learn to communicate effectively with this caring doctor on a regular basis.

The all around anti-hypertensive diet might be summed up in this way. Sodium intake is a major factor in raising blood pressure. Too much alcohol consumption along with smoking and unhealthy weight gain are factors in raising blood pressure. Try to maintain a cholesterol level below 200. Potassium, calcium, and magnesium all play roles in keeping blood pressure properly in line. A diet high in fiber is also

42

recommended for those with hypertension. Limit processed and restaurant foods and increase your fruit and vegetable intake. Eat fish twice a week or take an omega 3-fish supplement all will help reduce blood pressure. Vitamins C, E and B-3 are important nutrients for the entire cardiovascular system. High blood pressure is a most common disorder and a potentially dangerous one for all of us. Millions of Americans suffer this insidious disease perhaps thinking that it will go away on its own. This is not the case. So many of these insidious diseases if neglected simply get progressively worse over time. This silent killer can and will produce a number of serious physical ailments associated with it such as heart disease, kidney failure and even strokes.

So we have covered weight issues and blood pressure conditions both of which are ultimately and intimately related. Our next issue of a health nature is another basic health issue. One that like weight issues and blood pressure conditions are regularly ignored by the general public.

Chapter 4: Diabetes

Diabetes, as well as overweight and hypertension have reached serious proportions in our society. In the United States 25.8 million people have diabetes. According to the American Diabetes Association nearly 6 million people have undiagnosed diabetes. In 2010 about 1.9 million new cases were diagnosed in people 20 years of age or older. If this continues by 2050 1 of 3 US adults will have diabetes (www.cdc.gov). This section of the book will focus primarily on prediabetes and type II diabetes.

Diabetes is a disease where the body doesn't have enough insulin, or is unable to use the insulin or both. The pancreas makes insulin. Insulin allows the glucose molecule (sugar) to enter the cells and then is converted to energy for our body to use. There is an increase in blood glucose because the body of a diabetic is unable to bring the glucose from the blood into the cells.

There are three main types of diabetes, Type I, Type II and gestational diabetes. Type I diabetes is an autoimmune disease and is not preventable. It is first diagnosed in children or young adults. The treatment requires insulin. Type II diabetes accounts for 90-95% of all diabetes. It is associated with older age, obesity, physical inactivity, and family history of type II diabetes and history of gestational diabetes.

44

Gestational diabetes can develop during pregnancy when there is too much glucose in the blood. Soon after delivery the blood glucose levels returns to normal, but this increases your chances of developing Type II diabetes in the future.

Prediabetic individuals have a higher risk of developing type II diabetes. According to the CDC an estimated 79 million US adults had prediabetes in 2010. If you have been diagnosed with prediabetes you can still control your future. There are measures you can take. You can enroll in a prediabetes support group where you will learn healthy eating habits and ways to increase your physical activity level. They found that prediabetic adults who lost 5-7% of their body weight and had moderate physical activity 30 minutes for 5 days a week were able to reduce their risk of developing type II diabetes by 58%.

Symptoms of type II diabetes are often subtle. According to the Mayo Clinic here are some diabetes symptoms to look for, excessive thirst and increase urination, fatigue, weight loss, blurred vision, slow-healing sores or frequent infections, tingling hands and feet, and red, swollen, tender gums. If you are experiencing any of these conditions contact your doctor. Diabetes is a serious disordered and, if left untreated it can lead to heart disease, stroke, blindness, kidney failure, and amputations of feet and legs not related to accidents or injury. If diagnosed early then treatment will begin and you can lead a happy, healthy, longer life.

If you have been diagnosed with diabetes there are effective ways you can manage and control your diabetes. You are and will be in control! In healthy eating you should have a balance of carbohydrates, protein and fat (Mayo clinic). Your carbohydrates should consist of fruits, vegetables, and wholegrain pasta and bread. It is important that it has a low glycemic index. Glycemic index is the effect carbohydrates in food have on blood sugar levels. You should eat lean protein in the form of fish, white meat, milk, cheese, eggs, soy and beans. You must limit fat intake especially saturated fat. Choose low-fat or skim fat products and use low-fat vegetable cooking spray and don't fry food, rather bake, grill, or roast instead. It is vitally important that you discuss with your doctor or any other expert on your meal plans.

Physical activity is crucial in controlling diabetes. You should have 30 minutes of moderate physical activity 5 times a week. Moderate physical activity is when you have an increase in heart rate and breathing, and you should burn 3.5 to 7 calories per minute (Medical News Today). Always consult with your doctor before starting any exercise routine. Physical activity helps to control your blood glucose, helps you lose weight and/or maintain your weight, lowers and maintain your blood pressure, raises your HDL cholesterol (good cholesterol) and

46

lowers your LDL cholesterol (bad cholesterol) and improves your general mental health. Being a part of a gym and support group can help in achieving your treatment goals.

Diabetes is not a sentence to long-term disability or early death if you take personal control. Do have positive thoughts and attitudes towards managing your diabetes. Combined with healthy eating, increase physical activity, be a part of a support group and network and if necessary seek medication all this can help with controlling diabetes. YOU can lead a healthy life even with diabetes.

Chapter 5: Stress and Its Relationship to Your Health

When I was in my 50's I was under a lot of stress. I was working two jobs, married with three adult children, who at that time two were involved in the drug culture, my father had just passed away, and I was care taking my mother. One night I woke up with pressure on my chest. I was convinced I was experiencing a heart attack. My wife took me to the emergency room. I thought I was going to die. Fortunately, that was not the case. I was prescribed anxiety pills, told to contact my primary care physician and was released to go home. I saw my doctor and was informed that basically I was not in the best of shape. I was over-weight, my blood pressure was elevated, and I was prediabetic. That news was my big wake up call. I started taking care of myself by exercising on a regular basis and watching what I ate. It wasn't easy. I had my share of failed attempts, but I kept trying. Eventually with much help and support I was able to decrease my weight and normalize my blood pressure.

For all of us stress is in our everyday life. We cannot live without it. No one can live without experiencing some degree of stress. According to Hans Selyze an expert on stress and its management, in his book, The Stress of Life, he states that excess stress over time does come with difficulties of a more severe physical nature. Selyze states that one way excess stress causes illness is by destroying the body's immunological defense mechanisms. In other words too much stress stops the body's ability to fight off harmful diseases. For example, high level of adrenaline (epinephrine) and cortisol reduces our ability to rest and this cuts off needed sleep and often creates poor eating habits. True and helpful stress, the author continues is only good if it is short lived.

There are many causes of stress. Stress often results from anything that annoys you, threatens you, prods you, excites you, scares you, worries you, hurries you, angers you, and frustrates you. When you experience stress, your sympathetic nervous system sends a signal to your adrenal glands to secret adrenaline, this causes an increase heart rate to increase blood supply and increase respiratory rate for more oxygen and cortisol increases the production of glucose for the muscle to use. It mobilizes your body for fight or flight. When the stressor is gone then the body goes back to normal. Chronic stress tends to keep the body in the fight or flight state and the body is therefore unable to rest. Continual stress over time can lead to psychological, emotional and physical problems.

Stress is a risk factor for heart disease. Chronic stress increases the presence of stress hormones adrenaline and cortisol. There is abundant evidence to support the belief that excessive circulating adrenaline and cortisol lies behind many disease factors. Chronic stress can accelerate blood clots and atherosclerosis, increase blood pressure and elevate cholesterol, triglycerides and fatty acids.

A recent study made in June of 2003 edition of Stroke shows a connection between the severity of stress and induced blood pressure changes and strokes. A long-term Danish study had this finding. In this study it was determined that middle aged men who reported high levels of stress were as likely to suffer fatal strokes when compared to other men who reported low stress levels. It was shocking to find in this study that as little as one incident of stress a week could double the chance of a stroke.

As a medical doctor, my father, saw first hand stress related diseases. It is impossible to avoid stress completely, but he felt that if only his patients were able to follow his advice on managing chronic stress they could have added many years to their life.

There are effective ways to manage stress. Relaxation techniques such as deep breathing, yoga and meditation can often allow your body to return to a relaxed and rested state. Coping techniques such as setting realistic expectations for yourself, saying "no" when your plate is full, time management skills, exercising regularly, healthy eating and getting enough rest are all helpful. Having a more positive attitude will allow you to assess stressful situations more clearly. You can be objective about the situation, realize what can and cannot be changed and what your options may be.

Chapter 6: Medical Records and What They Can Tell Us

After my father's passing I found thousands of his medical records. My dad was a man trained in physical medicine but also saw the mental health issues carried by many of his patients. Often as a counseling psychologist I saw that he was most concerned and often perplexed by his patients and their lack of concern about their own health issues. Dr. Howe firmly believed that his patients could add another ten or twenty years to their life if they would listen and act on his well founded medical advice. I have selected a number of medical cases to see what we can learn from this well trained doctor.

A white female age 61 seeks medical advice because of numbness. She is rather unsteady with gout. She is an admitted chronic alcoholic with peripheral neuropathy and an enlarged liver. To date the patient is consuming large amounts of alcohol partly due to marital difficulties. She is advised strongly to discontinue her alcohol consumption. B12 is given. It is hoped she will follow Dr. Howe's advice. He believes that considerable recovery can be achieved by reformed alcoholics. A possible referral of this patient to Alcoholic Anonymous or a therapist is recommended.

Yet another patient is aged 64, have liver cirrhosis, a thrombosed hemorrhoid and an acute duodenal ulcer. It is noted here that at each of the doctor's visits real physical anomalies are found and follow up on the patient problems is done. As we have researched the doctor/patient records many of these cases reveal damaged organs due to the abusive use of alcohol. Probably primarily used to dull individual's emotional problems. We also see many health conditions are often brought on by poor dietary habits. That is mainly, due according to Dr. Howe by low fiber diets that are not conducive to good organ health.

A male patient aged 60 is diagnosed with rather severe rectal bleeding plus a right side hernia. This later condition is often formed in middle aged and older people who are out of shape and overweight. Additionally they also may have held to a low fiber diet.

A white female patient, age 53 has symptoms of type II diabetes. Patient is given blood test screening for diabetes. Results show she is positive for diabetes. During examination a lump was found in her left breast. Biopsy proves to be malignant. Radial mastectomy was performed. Good news no malignant cells were found in her glands. Seems to be adjusting well in the post treatment area.

The next patient has a series of problems. He has weakness in left thigh and is worried about a number of things. The odor of alcohol is present. He states that he has been drinking heavily. There is no atrophy of extremities but there is possible alcoholic neuropathy and cirrhosis of the liver. He was advised to stop drinking but he has not done. The patient's leg is getting weaker. It is recommended to the patient to initiate a high quality diet and multi-vitamins. This particular individual also smokes a pack of cigarettes a day. This type of patient is of a common variety found in our medical offices states Dr. Howe.

He has little awareness of his possible injury potentials. He fell off a porch recently while working and has a concentric hernia. He feels that these accidents, "Just happen." Being unaware of health realities can be quite a dangerous condition. The doctor believes he is close to being a medical disaster.

My father's general impression is that with good medical advice and treatment most people who take serious charge of their health should make it to the age of 85 without a great number of health abnormalities. Particularly if they are made aware of potential health issues on the horizon.

The next patient is a female age 64 admitted to the hospital with a history of severe anterior chest pains radiating into neck and arms for about 5 minutes in the mornings. This is probably coronary insufficiency. She had an early hysterectomy. Mother and sister had diabetes. No peripheral edema.

As our physician has indicated previously many if not most people in there sixties and seventies often have some heart difficulties. This is all the more reason to treat our heart with care and concern early on. With a proper diet, moderate exercise and weight control we will not have to wind up in the hospital prematurely.

Yet still another common condition, reflective of our modern, hectic society is illustrated by a male patient. He has protruding and bleeding hemorrhoids. His father died of a stroke at 73. Mother is still alive at 70. She has arthritis and heart disease. He frequently has headaches at night. There is also a polyp on his rectum. Too often patients such as this have intestinal problems too early on particularly since they often do not drink enough water and do not consume a proper high fiber diet. It is also important to remember that fruits and vegetables are a great source of fiber and do not contain any cholesterol. Animal foods and their by products contain cholesterol. Although our bodies do generate our own cholesterol we can control its effects by generating the good elements of cholesterol through proper exercise.

A person with a weight issue, age 43, has angina pain and blood pressure is 130/70. Heart tones are of a distant quality. No sign of murmurs present. He has been drinking quite a bit of coffee each day and smoking heavily. Dr. Howe tells the patient to discontinue all coffee consumption and cigarette smoking as soon as possible. A follow up visit will be necessary.

As can be seen changes in habits may bring one great health gains. The difficult thing is to eliminate or discontinue such ingrained bad habits. Both the doctor and patient together need to address these issues and come up with solutions. Simply to go "cold turkey" from a habit is not always a very successful strategy. Dr. Howe indicates follow up appointments for patients with such issues. Luckily medicine has recently improved ways to phase out smoking habits.

Another patient with many health symptoms at age 52 is well nourished and has had angina pectoris for the past 10 years. Angina pain is often controlled fairly well with use of medication plus nitroglycerine. Patient had a right femoral hernia repaired 7 years ago but it has since reoccurred. Father died in his 50's of coronary artery occlusion and heart failure. He has a 65 years old sister, who has angina pectoris. Another sister 54 years old who has heart disease and a brother 57 years old who had angina pectoris. It seems obvious that this patient has a family history with many, many examples of poor family health habits. These need to be explored and corrected by the doctor and patient in tandem.

This case is a female age 52, who now weighs 166 lbs as against earlier weight of 147 lbs. Also her blood pressure is 180/100, has overt chronic asthmatic bronchitis and hypertension. This patient often sighs a great deal and has trouble sleeping. This patient was operated on 10 years ago for acute diverticulitis of the sigmoid and a resection done with an end-to-end anastomosis. Colonoscopy shows presence of multiple

56

diverticulosis along the sigmoid. Father died at 68 from heart disease. Mother died at the age of 76 from heart disease. One sister died at 57 in her sleep.

Another common syndrome that is demonstrated by another patient is presented by a man of age 69 who has an enlarged heart. Lately he has been short of breath and is having severe coughing seizures. The patient is overweight. He additionally has been having some dizziness and instability. Dr. Howe feels he should go on a low calorie diet and the individual has indeed been losing weight. His blood pressure is 160/90, with abnormal EKG, Atrial flutter with AV (atrioventricular) block. Right bundle branch block.

The doctor's conclusion is mild cardiomegaly pulmonary vascular congestion and early pulmonary edema. As he states there are too many examples of this kind of patient who is overweight and has associated high blood pressure and heart problems. As has been indicated recently, overweight conditions have been more than obvious in our American society in recent times in fact even reaching near epidemic proportions in our population.

Another case is that of a female patient complaining of abdominal pain and tenderness. She has an enlarged liver. Through laboratory tests she was diagnosed with Alcoholic hepatitis, which is an inflammation of the liver, which the body's immune system responds to and causes liver damage. She is advised to discontinue all alcohol consumption. In addition the patient is diagnosis with gout, which is a form of arthritis. Lab studies from the blood uric acid test show an exceedingly elevated uric acid level of 12 mg/dl (normal range for women 2.4-6.0 mg/dl). Additionally she should also reduce her salt intake and increase water consumption, eat plenty of fruits, and eat limited amounts of chicken, pork and lean meat. As the doctor believes recovery by the human body can be marvelous if proper discipline is applied over time.

If the patient discontinues all alcohol it is possible to reverse the damage that has been done or in the least prevent the disease from becoming worse. Also it is recommended for the patient to have a special diet to reverse nutritional deficiencies that occur in people with alcoholic hepatitis. So, according to the doctor's analysis some positive health benefits may return with significant change in personal habits. Too often alcohol consumption can be seen as a failing attempt to mask problems in the patients personal life. This is one case where doctor's orders should be followed and reinforced with follow up doctor's appointments. This is a life or death medical prognosis. This case and several others do demonstrate the negative effects of the over use of alcohol which has a very negative effect on the human body.

Another common phenomena illustrated by the next two cases of injuries are results of automobile accidents. A male, age 40 was

58

involved in an accident. He sustained a flexion injury of the cervical spine. It has masked exacerbation of some existing nervousness and anxiety symptoms. He received physical therapy for the injury. Patient needed cervical traction and still has cervical muscle spasms and also neck pain and posterior occipital headache. He has been partially incapacitated since the time of the accident. Any stooping or bending will cause a rather marked exacerbation of his neck pain. He should however experience a complete recovery from the accident. He continues to improve but gradually.

Yet another auto accident victim is a 47-year-old white male. He has had jarring injury to head and neck and the lumbar and thoracic spine area remain as a result of injuries from this automobile accident. His car was hit from the rear by another car. If he is on his feet for a long time or holds his head still for any length of time he experiences vertigo. He also experiences urinary frequency and notes that he has to empty his bladder rather promptly. He had one sister who died as a result of injuries received in an automobile accident. This patient's symptoms will gradually subside and will probably not recur with any significant impairment although he may have some sensory impairment of the left hand and fingers for a considerable length of time.

Often many accident victims will take considerable time to heal properly. This of course is dependent on the severity of the accident.

Both this and the previous alcohol problem must be followed up medically to encourage patient recovery. Once again the human body does have great recovery potential in and of itself. The patient however does need additional help and encouragement in the slow recovery process he or she may be going through. There may be periods of depression, which should be recognized and treated as medical issues.

Another patient, female age 73 admitted to the hospital because of a fall at home and was unable to get up. She has severe ulceration of the right leg, a history of frequent and incontinent stools and is drinking alcohol to an excess. On admission patient had systolic and diastolic murmurs, an enlarged liver, enlarged spleen, an ulcer of the right leg and a rapid irregular pulse with some atrial fibrillation. Started on Digoxin (used to treat congestive heart failure and to slow the heart rate in patients with atrial fibrillation) soon lapsed into congestive heart failure. Ulcer on leg became worse. A rather grim analysis but as Dr. Howe has said on occasion he has seen patients live who should have died and those who died who should have lived. A suddenly disciplined life and a will to live can do much for the recovery process.

Another interesting case is of a female nurse, age 73 who had hypertension for many years until the last couple of years at which time it seemed to be down to normal levels and running between 160/90 to 150/80. In addition to this she has had gout over the past 4 or 5 years and has had several attacks of this high uric acid running 10 mg/dl. She has an irregular heart beat indicating some fibrillation problems. Also 12 years ago had a bilateral vein stripping done at the hospital. Father died at age 55 of an accident, mother died at age 73 of carcinoma of the stomach. She had 8 brothers and sisters, all of whom have passed away, one of tuberculosis, one of a malignancy and the rest probably cardiac arrest (the heart develops an arrhythmia that causes the heart to stop beating, this is different from a heart attack, where the heart usually continues to beat but the blood flow to the heart is blocked). The patient has a great deal of trouble with walking because of weakness and pain in her joints of her legs. Heart is absolutely irregular and somewhat difficult to hear, 120 beats/minute.

Looking at this patient's record we can see a family history of medical problems that are evident and expressed in this patient. Probably there is an overuse of alcohol as a factor and also the stress involved in her occupation. Many of these patients previously mentioned have had a history of alcohol use or abuse, which could have damaged their biological systems. Cessation of alcohol use can or should have been helpful in their recovery. It should be remembered that alcohol is a neurotoxin and its abuse could lead to long-term disastrous results.

As we go through the doctor's patient records we see so many cases of damaged organs due mainly to the abuse of alcohol. Often people see alcohol as an escape from pain or from a feeling of emptiness or depression. Temporarily it dulls the pain; it certainly will not lessen the problem issues in their life. The doctor may offer psychological help, nutrition information, and exercise routines that alleviate the patient from the abuse of alcohol, depression or mood swings. Too often patient will discover that they have just fallen into another health entrapment of their own making.

Additionally we also see a common condition brought on by poor dietary habits. One condition is diverticulosis. Diverticulosis is very common. It is found in half of Americans over the age of 60. Diverticulosis is a condition that develops when pouches form in the wall of the large intestine. It is not completely understood what causes these pouches.

Doctors think these pouches form when high pressure pushes against weak spots in the colon wall. When there is adequate amount of fiber in the diet, bulky soft stool is formed and easily moves through the colon. If there is not enough fiber then small hard stool is formed and increases the time the stool is in the intestines thus adding pressure. Diverticulitis occurs when there is an infection in the pouches.

What is learned from reviewing the numerous medical records

besides the health diagnosis, we find the importance of knowing family health history and the physical and mental impact health has on the patient. Dr. Howe indicates older patients often signal serious depression when dealing with many of these chronic health issues. It is important for physicians, families and friends to be supportive of the patient. It is equally important for the patient to examine their own health patterns as well as their family health histories and discuss them with their doctor in some detail.

Chapter 7: Exercise and Related Issues

An expert in the field of exercise and fitness is Dr. George Sheehan. He was a long term practicing cardiologist out of my dad's era. What made Dr. Sheehan unique is that he renewed his life at the age of 45 through running and he shared his experience with the world. He wrote a column in a local newspaper for 25 years, served as a medical editor for Runner's World Magazine, gave lectures and wrote 8 books.

He has often sadly stated that only some 10% of Americans exercise up to recommended medical guidelines. Most doctors want their patients to exercise on a regular basis. Americans he believes seem unwilling to obey the rules for fitness except when it comes to giving up their couch potato sedentary lifestyles.

Sheehan states that joggers and cyclists for example represent but a limited proportion of the American public, which for the most part remain sedentary. Dr. Sheehan states that the importance of exercise to a long and productive life is only too evident. He states emphatically that the US population's heart attack rate double that of most European countries. This despite the fact that we are more observant of smoking cessation and diet routines. This leads to the deciding factor in the heart attack dilemma, which is a lack of proper and consistent exercise. He continues that a high drop out rate in fitness programs further reveals this deciding factor, which is appalling.

According to Sheehan almost 70% of exercise starters backslide into a sedentary lifestyle. Consistency he believes is a vital component to a successful exercise program. He further believes decisively that in order for fitness programs to be successful, people must enjoy the exercise so that they will stick with it over time.

To support his contention about the importance of exercise he believes that well conditioned individuals rate higher than unconditioned persons in emotional stability, sensitivity and diminished anxiety.

Fitness according to Sheehan is simply the ability to do work and induce in your workout time a period for stretching, as well. In your training routine you should consume sufficient amounts of water. Stay hydrated. This cardiologist further states that by middle age more than 50% of Americans are overweight and hate their condition. Unknowingly they have doubled their risk of heart disease, triple their chances of having gallstones and increased by four times their incidence of Type II diabetes. Sadly too often attempts to diet lead to failure. Sheehan continues to state that the body fat lost in fad diets often return to individuals.

In conjunction with diet and exercise is the rational, scientific and successful way to lose weight permanently. In his study of runners,

Sheehan found, as a group runners are rarely overweight or over fat. Sheehan is a strong believer in running, jogging and strong walking as exercise. It is so easy to do. As one of my former bosses stated, "I like this type of exercise. It is easy for me to put on my running shoes and go for a fitness run or walk."

A brilliant doctor from Harvard Medical School once told me, "Bob, keep running and when you can not run any longer then jog and when you can no longer jog then walk." I have followed his advice and after many years my cardiovascular condition has been excellent. Many of my friends who did not maintain an exercise routine have either died or have had heart related issues and had to undergo surgery or sometimes multiple surgeries.

Sheehan continues that exercise affords important metabolic benefits. The blood lipid profile approaches the ideal. Total cholesterol and triglycerides go down and high-density lipoproteins (HDL) go up, glucose tolerance improves, insulin levels decrease, blood pressure drops thus improving your overall health and fitness level.

Such positive results of running and indeed of any aerobic exercise program (swimming, biking, hiking, walking, etc) make exercise a most rational and scientific choice particularly for overweight people. Of course you should check your fitness level with your doctor before embarking on a strong exercise program.

In Sheehan's personal program, he runs at a comfortable level so he can observe the world around him. At that pace he feels he forgets he is running and he does just 45 minutes to an hour. At his speed running becomes automatic. It has the same health effects as swimming he feels.

Sheehan has a well-made finishing point. He has a friend who teaches a fitness course. His students lift weights one day and jog the next but they rarely drop out of his class. Why? Well, because the daily workouts are all part of a mountain-climbing course that prepares all 25 students to climb Oregon's Mt. Hood.

I as the author have a similar focus. I lift weights one day and the next day I do a cardiovascular workout. My long-term goal is to participate in the Senior Olympics. Having some goals in your exercise program can help you to stay motivated and focused in your chosen exercise routine!

As a related issue to that of the fitness issue are those of the heart. Heart rhythm problems can be serious and should be monitored. Such issues can cause fainting, shortness of breath and chest pain. This can put you at high risk for heart failure and even strokes of various kinds! This can be treated by medications. Doctors may prescribe beta-blockers and channel calcium blockers to help control an irregular heart rate. Blood thinners may be prescribed to reduce the risk of blood clots and strokes in the circulatory system. You should discuss all medications you are taking with your physician to decrease possible adverse drug interactions.

Swimming is an excellent exercise. Swimming has been found to reduce blood pressure and improve artery health in adults according to a study in the American Journal of Cardiology. Additionally, swimming puts less stress on joints than other forms of exercise. Researchers tested 43 adults from 50 to 80 years of age. All had pre-hypertension conditions but otherwise healthy. One group swam 15 to 45 minutes a day, 3 to 4 days a week for 12 weeks. The control group spent time stretching and learning relaxation exercise. They found the swimming group blood pressure went from 131mmHg to 122mmHg. This is a 7% decrease on the blood pressure reading. The arteries also showed signs of becoming more elastic and responsive to changes in blood flow. The swimming group did not lose any weight or fat. The control group showed no statistically significant improvements.

The researchers felt that the trial group should continue their workouts and that this would decrease their risk of heart disease significantly. It is also important to keep your bones strong. Your skeletal system is your support system. Osteoporosis is a condition that causes our bones to become brittle which often leads to bones breaking more easily. Bone density decreases with age and more women than men develop this disease.

Food high in calcium such as milk, cheese, and yogurt contain forms of calcium your body absorbs readily. Additionally dark green vegetables, beans, dried fruits and nuts and fortified cereals and juices also provide calcium, which helps to strengthen your bone structure.

In conjunction to calcium intake your exercise routine walking and weight lifting should help improve your bone structure. If bones are weakened, falls can produce severe injuries. Strong bones protect you against this possibility. As a personal example, I recently fell and hit the ground hard. Fortunately I sustained a few bruises and no broken bones. This is because I lift weights regularly, 3 times a week, and cardio exercise, the days I don't lift weight, to build a strong skeletal system and a healthy body.

Chapter 8: What it Means to be Over 50

Fifty sneaks up on you. Before you know it you are celebrating your 50th birthday and beyond. You wonder where did the time go? You have been so busy building a career and raising a family. You think of 50 and beyond as a time when everything goes down hill. Stop thinking that way. Rather think this is going to be the best time of my life.

As mentioned in the previous chapters there may be health issues that you will have to soon face. There is however an abundance of helpful information available to you. Inform yourself so that you can make the best decision for yourself and your body. I have repeated over and over again in this book, the mantra that you control what and how much you eat and your activity level. I believe this is a major key to healthy living.

Eating in a healthy fashion is important to your overall well being. Choose food wisely that helps to lower your blood cholesterol and which decreases your risk of heart disease. This includes foods low in fat, low in cholesterol (mainly animal products); increase dietary fiber intake and decrease salt and alcohol intake and increase water consumption.

Most people are normally in a chronically dehydrated state. Even mildly dehydrated you can experience headaches and it may make you feel tired. You need to be properly hydrated. Water makes up more than 60% of our body weight, our brain is made up of about 75% water, blood is about 80% and our lungs are about 80%. Therefore adequate water is needed to maintain a proper blood volume. Water regulates our body temperature, removes harmful toxins from our body, and transports nutrients (via the blood). Fundamentally our body needs water to function properly.

How much water should we drink? According to the Mayo Clinic the adequate intake for men is roughly 3 liters (about 13 cups) and for women 2.2 liters (about 9 cups) of total beverages a day. There are other fluid sources such as what you eat, like fruits and vegetables. There are factors that influence water consumption such as exercise, environment, and illnesses or health conditions. As a rule if you produce 1.5 liters (6.3 cups) of colorless or light yellow urine a day and you rarely feel thirsty then you are probably drinking enough fluids. You should check with your doctor to determine the correct amount of water that is right for you.

There are many fad diets in the market today. Avoid them instead eat quality whole foods, fruits and vegetables, whole grains, lean meat and fresh fish. Stay clear of processed foods. They are high in cholesterol, fat and salt. Monitor the quantity of food. Portion control is a vital key. A helpful online resource from the USDA is www.choosemyplate.gov. This web page has a wealth of current information to assist you in making healthy food choices and it has a very useful tool, SuperTracker, that helps you plan, analyze, and track your diet and physical activity.

Physical activity is most important. Fitness opens up the circuits in the amazing storage and retrieval system that is our human brain. It gives us another form of energy that is the willpower that comes with discipline and the ascetic life style. Fitness is movement and energy not only muscular but also cognitive.

Doctors have found fitness fights disease on two fronts. It reduces life threatening physical risk factors and it reduces harmful psychological dilemmas such as hostility, tension, stress and anxiety that often beset us. Another benefit is that it improves your sleep.

Exercise has other important metabolic benefits. The blood lipid profile appears positive, the total cholesterol and triglycerides go down, HDL goes up, glucose tolerance improves, insulin levels decrease, blood pressure drops-all reducing the potential threat to our heart health. These physical and physiological results of running and strong walking or any aerobic exercise program, are the only rational and scientific choices for overweight people. Do include stretching exercises in your exercise routine. Stretching improves our flexibility. Flexibility helps to increase our range of motion and reduces our chance of injury when exercising and doing everyday activities. Furthermore, when you feel stronger and trimmer, this generally helps your self-image and self-esteem.

You may be thinking, "How do I start an exercise routine?" First step is to check with your doctor before starting your exercise routine. The advantage of an exchange with your physician is that it can help you find a program that matches your particular level of fitness.

In exercise you need to ask what type of exercise best fits you. Normally exercise can be broken down into three basic types: First, stretching or the slow lengthening and stretching of the muscles. Stretching before and after exercising helps prepare the muscles before activity and after. Stretching helps prevent injury and muscle strain. Secondarily, cardiovascular or aerobic exercise is a steady physical activity using large muscle groups. This type of exercise strengthens the heart and lungs and improves your body's ability to use oxygen. Lastly strengthening exercises, which empowers your muscle groups and strengthens your overall body. Exercise session should also include a warm up, conditioning phase and a cool down.

How can you avoid over doing your exercise program? You should gradually increase your activity level, especially if you have not been exercising regularly. You should also wait at least one and a half hrs after eating a meal before exercising. Additionally you should take time to include a 5-minute warm-up including stretching exercises, then your aerobic activity and then include a five to ten minute cool down after the activity phase. Try also to keep an exercise record of your progress over time.

Whether you are under 50 or over, remember it is never too early or late to enhance your health to a state of excellence. This book contains the wisdom of medical research and of a wise old physician and should take you down the road to a state of well balance health. As my dad so concretely stated to me in our frequent discussions on longevity, "Bob, if some of my patients would only listen to me I could put 10 to 20 years additionally on their lives." He might have added, "Read this book like a bible and you will never regret a healthy life well lived."

www.ingramcontent.com/pod-product-compliance
Lightning Source LLC
Chambersburg PA
CBHW020354290526
45785CB00005B/2276